Nour Elleuch
Ahmad Youssfi
Wafa Dahmani

Upper gastrointestinal bleeding in non-cirrhotic portal cavernoma

Nour Elleuch
Ahmad Youssfi
Wafa Dahmani

Upper gastrointestinal bleeding in non-cirrhotic portal cavernoma

Associated factors

ScienciaScripts

Imprint

Cover image: www.ingimage.com

This book is a translation from the original published under ISBN 978-620-6-73045-3.

Publisher:
Sciencia Scripts
is a trademark of
Dodo Books Indian Ocean Ltd. and OmniScriptum S.R.L publishing group

120 High Road, East Finchley, London, N2 9ED, United Kingdom
Str. Armeneasca 28/1, office 1, Chisinau MD-2012, Republic of Moldova, Europe
Managing Directors: Ieva Konstantinova, Victoria Ursu
info@omniscriptum.com

Printed at: see last page
ISBN: 978-620-8-64564-9

FACTORS ASSOCIATED WITH THE OCCURRENCE UPPER GASTROINTESTINAL HAEMORRHAGE DUE TO PORTAL HYPERTENSION IN NON-CIRRHOTIC PORTAL CAVERNOMA

INTRODUCTION

Chronic portal vein thrombosis without underlying liver disease, also known as non-cirrhotic portal cavernoma, is defined by the appearance of a network of tortuous collateral veins around the portal trunk after prolonged obstruction in a healthy liver(1) . This condition is the leading cause non-cirrhotic portal hypertension (PH) in Western countries (2,3). The clinical presentation of non-cirrhotic portal cavernoma is generally marked by the occurrence of PH complications dominated varicose upper gastrointestinal haemorrhage. Digestive haemorrhage due to PH is the most frequent complication during follow-up patients with non-cirrhotic portal cavernoma. Its high morbidity and mortality make it a formidable complication. However, published data are scarce (4). To our knowledge, Tunisian study has been published on this subject. In our work, we set out to identify the factors associated with the occurrence of digestive haemorrhage due to PH in patients with non-cirrhotic portal cavernoma.

PATIENTS AND METHODS

I- MATERIALS :

We conducted a single-centre retrospective cross-sectional study in the gastroenterology department of Sahloul University Hospital, over a 10-year period from January 2010 to December 2019.

1- INCLUSION :

All non-cirrhotic patients over the age of 18 with portal cavernoma were included in our study. The diagnosis of chronic portal thrombosis was based on the absence of flow in the portal vein and the visualisation of a network of porto-portal collateral shunts corresponding to the cavernoma on abdominal Doppler ultrasound or 4-stage contrast-enhanced cross-sectional imaging (CECI).

2- NON-INCLUSION CRITERIA :

Our study did not include all patients with thrombosis related to cirrhosis or hepatocellular carcinoma.

3- EXCLUSION CRITERIA :

Our study did not include :

▸ Patients hospitalisation or consultation records could not be used or could not be found.

▶ Patients with <3 months follow-up.

II - METHOD :

1-DATA COLLECTION :

A pre-established data collection form **(Appendix I)** was completed for all patients, and the following data were collected:

1-1. Socio-demographic and anamnestic data :

▶ Age

▶ The genre

▶ Tobacco consumption quantified in annual packets

▶ Alcohol consumption. In the case of excessive consumption (>20 g/d for women and >30 g/d for men), average consumption was quantified (in grams of alcohol per day).

▶ Personal medical history of thromboembolic venous pathology, of diabetes, , ischaemic heart disease and dyslipidaemia.

▶ Personal history of visceral surgery, intra-abdominal infection, abdominal trauma, acute pancreatitis, or relapse of chronic inflammatory bowel disease in the 3 months preceding the diagnosis of portal cavernoma.

▶ Gynaeco-obstetric history and use of oral contraceptives.

▸ A known family history of venous thrombosis or thrombophilia.

▸ The circumstances in which the is discovered.

▸ The time between the first symptoms and diagnosis.

1-2. Clinical data

▸ The presence of signs of PH (splenomegaly, collateral venous circulation type porto-cava, ascites)

▸ The presence of and abdominal tenderness.

1-3. Biological data

The following data were collected for each patient:

A standard biological work-up including :

- Blood count (CBC): haemoglobin (Hb), haematocrit, platelets (elements/mm^3) and white blood cells (elements/mm^3).
- Renal assessment. ionogram, blood urea and creatinine levels.
- Liver function tests: aspartate amino transferase (ASAT), alanine amino transferase (ALAT), gamma-glutamyl transferase (GGT), alkaline phosphatase (ALP), total and conjugated bilirubin BT and BC), prothrombin rate (PT) and International Normalized Ratio (INR).
- Serum protein electrophoresis.

A thrombophilia work-up including :

- Measurement of activated Protein C (PC)by chronometric method. Patients with an activated PC ≤ 70% were considered PC deficient.

- Protein S assay using the chronometric method. Patients with a ≤ 55% were considered to be protein S deficient.

- The search for a factor V mutation and/or resistance to activated PC by chronometric method. We considered that plasmas with a clotting time ≤ 120 s were resistant to activated PC.

- The search a factor II mutation

- Antithrombin (AT) levels. Patients with a level <80% were considered deficient in TA.

- Testing for anti-phospholipid syndrome by measuring anti-cardiolipin antibodies and anti-β-2Glycoprotein I antibodies using enzyme-linked immunosorbent assay techniques and circulating lupus-type anticoagulant antibodies using chronometric techniques.
- Determination of plasma homocysteine levels by chromatographic method, after fasting for 12 hours (usual values: 5 to 15 µmol/l) and, if applicable, a mutation of the methyl tetrahydrofolate reductase (MTHFR) gene.

- Search for Paroxysmal Nocturnal Haemoglobinuria by flow cytometry or Ham-Dacie test

- The search a myeloproliferative syndrome by looking for the JAK 2. If positive, an osteo-medullary biopsy was performed.

1-4.Endoscopic data

All patients oeso-gastro-duodenal endoscopy (EOGD) within the first year of treatment. as part of the PH .
The following were specified:

▶ The presence or absence of oesophageal varices (OV). They are classified according to the classification proposed by the Japanese Research Society for Portal Hypertension, which has been modified by the New Italian Endoscopic Club into 3 grades according to the size of the varices (5).

▶ The presence or absence of gastric varices. Gastric varices are classified according to their location using the Sarin classification(6).

▶ The presence or absence of hypertensive gastropathy. The diagnosis of hypertensive gastropathy was made in the presence a mosaic appearance and was classified according to the NIEC classification (7).

▶ The presence or absence of severe PH. Endoscopic portal hypertension was considered severe in the presence of VO grade II or III, gastric varices or severe hypertensive gastropathy (4).

1.5. Radiological data :

All patients underwent 4-stage injected cross-sectional imaging.
The following were specified:
-The partial or total nature of the portal thrombosis, its extent and extension upstream to the splanchnic vessels (splenic vein, superior mesenteric vein) and downstream (intra-hepatic portal branches).

- The presence of signs of PH.

- The presence of associated complications such as ischaemia or mesenteric infarction, ascites and biliary complications.

- Elements that may help in making an aetiological diagnosis (the presence of deep-seated neoplasia, pancreatic pathology .....)

If portal cholangiopathy was suspected, cholangio-MRI was performed.

1.6. Aetiological diagnosis :

All patients a comprehensive aetiological work-up. This included a search for of:

- ▶ A local cause
- ▶ A thrombophilia factor
- ▶ Myeloproliferative syndrome
- ▶ Search other factors: search for neoplasia, disease, etc.

systemic (Behçet, coeliac disease...)

- ▶ Taking oral contraceptives or a recent pregnancy.

1.7. Evolution :

The duration of follow-up was defined as the time interval between the occurrence of the portal cavernoma and the date of the last consultation, the date of occurrence a digestive haemorrhage, the date of death, or the date of the end of our study. All patients were contacted by telephone. They were asked about the date of the last consultation or the date of death (by relatives). The duration, frequency and methods of clinical, biological and radiological follow-up were specified. The outcome of each patient was specified:

- Radiological evolution (stability, extension or partial or total repermeabilisation) spontaneously or under anticoagulant treatment.

- The occurrence of digestive or extra-digestive haemorrhagic complications with anti coagulation, their time of onset in relation to the start of treatment and their evolution.

1.8. Therapeutic methods :

Each a treatment for portal cavernoma was instituted, it was specified:
- The indication for treatment, type of anticoagulant treatment started and the total duration of treatment.

- Treatment PH :

○ In patients with large VO (grade II and III) or gastric varices, primary prophylaxis with non-cardioselastic B-Blockers or endoscopic oesophageal variceal ligation (EVLT) was introduced. The choice of one of the two therapeutic options was specified.

○ In the event of haemorrhage due to variceal rupture, vasoactive treatment and LEVO sessions in the event of VO rupture or an injection of biological glue in the event of LV rupture were inserted. Anticoagulant treatment was only reintroduced once the varicose veins had been eradicated.

- Aetiological treatment.

2- Statistical analysis :

The data was entered SPSS version 21 software. It comprised two sections: the first descriptive and the second analytical.

2-1. Descriptive study

For quantitative variables, we used averages and standard deviations and range (minimum value - maximum value). For qualitative variables, simple frequencies (numbers) and relative frequencies (percentages) were calculated.

2-2. Analytical study

The aim of our analytical study was to identify the factors associated with the occurrence of digestive haemorrhage due to PH. We compared the 2 groups of patients: with and without the occurrence of a digestive haemorrhage in order to identify the factors associated with its occurrence. The search for associated variables was first carried out by a univariate study, using Student's t-test for quantitative variables and Pearson's chi-square test and Fisher's exact test for qualitative variables, then completed by a multivariate analysis using logistic regression in order to identify the factors independently associated with the occurrence of digestive haemorrhage due to PH. For all statistical tests, the significance level was set at 0.05.

III. BIBLIOGRAPHICAL RESEARCH

A bibliographic search was carried out using scientific databases: Science Direct and Pub Med. The references were cited and managed by the ZOTERO software.

IV. ETHICAL CONSIDERATIONS

There were no conflicts of interest in this work. The confidentiality of individual data was respected throughout the study. Data were pseudonymised and only one investigator knew the identity of the patients. Given the retrospective nature of study, it was not possible to obtain informed consent from patients.

RESULTS

I. DESCRIPTIVE STUDY :

1. STUDY POPULATION :

In total, we studied 83 files of patients followed for a portal cavernoma over a period of 10 years. We did not include 32 cirrhotic patients and 2 patients with HCC. excluded 2 patients whose records could not be analysed. In the end, 47 cases were selected (Figure 1).

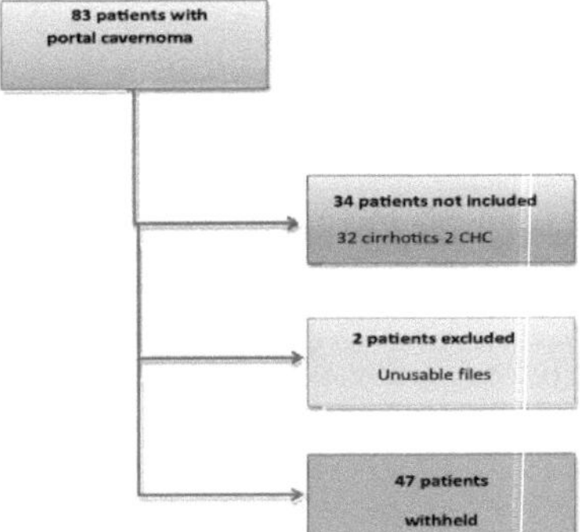

Figure 1: Study population

2. AGE

The average age of our patients was 40.7 years, with extremes ranging from 19 to 75 years. The age range between 20 and 40 was the most frequently reported (45%).

3. SEX

There were 24 women (51%) and 23 men (49%), with a sex ratio (male/female) of 0.95.

4. PERSONAL HISTORY:

4.1. Medical history :

The various medical histories are summarised in Table I.

	Table I: Medical history	
History	Number (N)	Percentage (%)
Hypertension	4	8,5
Diabetes	6	12,7
Dyslipidemia	4	8,5
Renal insufficiency	2	4,2
chronicle Vascular accident	2	4,2
ischaemic Celiac disease	1	2,1
Total	19	40,4

4.2. Surgical history :

A history of abdominal surgery was noted in 7 patients (14.8%). The mean time from diagnosis to surgery was 7.2 months, with extremes ranging from 1 to 16 months. The various interventions are detailed in Table II.

Table II: Surgical history

Interventions	Number (N)	Percentage (%)
Resection of the projecting dome of a	1	2,1
hydatid cyst of the liver Inguinal hernia repair	1	2,1
Umbilical hernia repair	1	2,1
Cholecystectomy	3	6,3
Splenectomy	1	2,1
Total	7	14,8

5. Clinical data

5.1. Start mode

time between diagnosis of the portal cavernoma and the onset of symptoms was less than two weeks in 6 cases (13%), between 2 weeks and one month in 4 cases (8%), and between one month and 3 months in 8 cases (17%). In 29 cases (62%), the delay was more than 3 months.

5.2. Reasons for consultation

Abdominal pain was the most frequent reason for consultation in 32 cases: the site was the epigastrium or right hypochondrium in 25 cases (78%), the pain was right lumbar in 3 cases and in the right iliac fossa in one case. Pain was diffuse in 3 cases (9%). The intensity was moderate in all cases. Incidental finding was reported in 9 cases (19%).The circumstances in which portal cavernoma is discovered are summarised in Table III.

Table III: Circumstances in which portal cavernoma is discovered

Circumstances of discovery	Number	Percentage
	(N)	(%)
Abdominal pain	32	68,1
Impaired general condition	10	21,3
Bleeding digestive by	9	19,1
portal hypertension		
Abdominal distension	2	4,3
Asymptomatic	9	19,1

5.3. Physical examination data:

The most frequent clinical signs were porto-cava collateral venous circulation in 24 patients (51.1%) and splenomegaly in 20 cases (42.5%). Hepatomegaly was present in 20 patients (42.5%).

6. Biological data:

Hepatic cytolysis was present in 6 cases (12%). Cholestasis was noted in 12 patients (25%). Renal failure was noted in 3 patients (6%). Anaemia was noted in 19 patients (40%). Hyperleukocytosis was present in 6 cases (13%) and thrombocytopenia in 9 cases (19%). The various biological parameters are summarised in Table IV.

	Table IV: Biological data	
Biological parameter	average± standard deviation	Extreme values
	or median [IIQ]	
ASAT (UI/L)	25 [20-30]	10-330
ALT (IU/L)	23 [16-26]	12-490
PAL (IU/L)	98 [75-150]	42-620
GGT (UI/L)	26 [16-62]	11-190
BT (μmol/L)	17 [12-16]	7-257
BD (μmol/L)	5 [2-9]	1-146
TP (%)	81±13	60-100
Urea (mmol/L)	4,8 [3,6-6]	2-25,1
Creatinine (μmol/L)	66 [55-76]	21-193
Na (mmol/L)	137,3±3,5	125-145
K (mmol/L)	4,1±0,4	3-5,3
CRP (mg/L)	6 [2-22]	1-180
Hb (g/dL)	12,2 [10-13,8]	5,6-16
GB (elements /μL)	7879±2891,6	3003-13870
Platelets (elements /μL)	207000 [147000-277000]	18100-870000
IQR: interquartile range		

7. Radiological data at time of diagnosis :

7.1. Type of additional examination :

Abdominal Doppler ultrasound was performed as the first-line examination in 41 patients (87%) and abdominal CT angiography in 6 patients (13%). All patients who underwent abdominal Doppler ultrasound in the first instance had their diagnosis confirmed by cross-sectional imaging with contrast medium injection.Seven patients (15%) further exploration using MRI.

7.2. Extension of thrombosis :

Total obstruction of the portal trunk was noted in all patients. In 14 patients (29%) thrombosis was limited to the portal trunk.

Downstream extension of the thrombosis to the right and left portal branches was noted in 20 cases (42%). Nine patients (19%) had exclusively downstream extension.Upstream extension to the splanchnic vessels was observed in 20 patients (42.5%). This is summarised in Table V. Extension to the superior mesenteric vein was noted in 15 patients (31%). One case of simultaneous thrombosis of the suprahepatic veins was noted.

Table V: Distribution according to the site of extension to the splanchnic vessels

Location of extension		**Number (N)**	**Percentage (%)**	
Door trunk		14	29,8	
Superior mesenteric vein (SMV)		**11**	**23,4**	
Splenic vein (SV)		3	6,4	
Spleno-mesenteric trunk (SMT)		1	2,1	
VMS+VS		3	6,4	
VMS+TSM		1	2,1	
TSM+VS		1	2,1	
Total		34	72	
VMS: Superior mesenteric vein mesaraic	VS:	Splenic vein	,TSM: Trunk	splen o-

7.3. Radiological signs of PH:

Splenomegaly was observed in 20 patients (42%). Collateral venous circulation (perigastric, perisplenic, mesenteric) was noted in 24 patients (51.1%). Moderate ascites was found in 2 patients. Repermeabilisation of the umbilical vein was observed in 23 patients (48.9%). The various radiological signs of PH are summarised in Table VI.

Table VI: Radiological signs portal hypertension

Signs radiological	Number	Percentage
PH	(N)	(%)
Splenomegaly	20	42,5
HVAC	24	51,1
Ascites	2	4,2
Rewaterproofing of the umbilical vein	23	48,9

CVC: collateral venous circulation , PH: portal hypertension

8. Endoscopic data :

EOGD was performed in all patients at the time of diagnosis. Twenty-nine patients (61%) had endoscopic evidence of PH. OVs were found in 23 patients (48.9%), with grade I OVs in 15 cases, grade II OVs in 3 cases and grade III OVs in 5 cases. No patient had a LV. Eighteen patients (38.2%) had hypertensive gastropathy, considered severe in 6 cases.

9. Etiological investigation :

The aetiological investigation did not identify an obvious cause of portal cavernoma in 19 cases (40.4%). Elsewhere, the cause was multiple in 4 patients (8.5%). Table VII summarises the different aetiologies of portal cavernoma.

Table VII: Results of aetiological assessment

Causes	Number	Percentage
	(N)	(%)
Prothrombotic states	11	23,4
hereditary		
Protein C deficiency	5	10,6
Protein S deficiency	1	2,1
Hyperhomocysteinemia	5	10,6
Prothrombotic states	10	21,2
acquired		
Essential thrombocythemia	1	2,1
Polyglobulia vaquez	1	2,1
SAPL	2	4,2
Celiac disease	2	4,2
Oral contraception	1	2,1
Post-partum	1	2,1
Behçet's disease	1	2,1
Lung cancer	1	2,1
metastatic		
Local cause	3	6,3
Hydatid cyst	1	2,1
Acute lithiasis pancreatitis	1	2,1
Pancreatic cancer	1	2,1
Linked causes	4	8,4
Hyperhomocysteinemi+	2	4,2
SAPL		
Essential thrombocythemia	1	2,1
+ SAPL		
Chronic pancreatitis	1	2,1
calcifying+ Deficiency in		
Protein C		
Undetermined cause	19	40,4
Total	47	100

SAPL: Antiphospholipid antibody syndrome

10. COMPLICATIONS :

Mean follow-up was 52.6 months [3-105 months].

Complications were found in 24 cases (50.).

10.1. Varicose digestive haemorrhage:

Digestive haemorrhage due to PH occurred in 16 patients (34%) during follow-up, with a delay of 22.3 months (range: 1-76 months). This was HDH due to rupture of the VO in the all cases. Seven patients (14.8%) were taking anticoagulants, 2 of whom were overdosing at the time of HDH.

10.2. Other complications:

The various complications are summarised in Table VIII.

Table VIII: Complications occurring during follow-up

Complications	Number (N)	Percentage (%)
Digestive haemorrhage	16	34
Portal cholangiopathy	7	14,8
Mesenteric ischaemia	1	2,1
Total	24	50,9

11. THERAPEUTIC DATA :

11.1. Anticoagulant treatment:

Anticoagulation was prescribed in 29 patients (61.7%). The duration of anticoagulant treatment was 54 months (range: 3-135 months).

11.2. Treatment of the underlying disease:

Patients with SMP were managed in collaboration with haematologists and started on hydroxycarbamide. In the two cases of metastatic cancer, with pulmonary and pancreatic primaries, palliative chemotherapy was introduced.

The patient presented with a calcified and compressive hydatid cyst and underwent surgery. Imaging showed no repermeabilisation of the portal trunk.

A patient Behçet's disease was treated with colchicine.
The 2 patients coeliac disease were put on a gluten-free diet.

11.3. Treatment hypertension

Beta-blockers were prescribed in 21 patients (44.6%) as primary prophylaxis in 8 cases and secondary prophylaxis in 13 cases.LEVO was performed in 18 patients (38.2%) as primary prophylaxis in 5 cases and secondary prophylaxis in 13 cases.In 10 cases (21%), it was carried out before the patient was started on anti-coagulants.

12. Mortality :

Overall mortality in our series was 10.6% (N=5).
The different causes of death are summarised in table IX.

	Table IX: Causes of death	
Cause of death	Number	Percentage
	(N)	(%)
Varicose haemorrhage	2	4,2
Mesenteric ischaemia	1	2,1
Severe acute angiocholitis	1	2,1
Pulmonary embolism	1	2,1
Total	5	10,6

II. ANALYTICAL STUDY: FACTORS ASSOCIATED WITH THE OCCURRENCE OF DIGESTIVE HAEMORRHAGE DUE TO HTP:

As previously indicated, the groups were split as follows:

- Group 1: included patients without variceal haemorrhage during follow-up (N=31)
- Group 2: included patients with variceal haemorrhage during follow-up (N=16)

The various parameters (epidemiological, clinical, biological and evolutionary) were compared between the two groups.

2.1. Univariate study :

2.1.1. Comparison of epidemiological characteristics

In univariate analysis, age and gender were not identified as factors associated with occurrence of digestive haemorrhage due to HTP.

Table X: Comparison of epidemiological characteristics in the occurrence of digestive haemorrhage due to PH

Digestive haemorrhage n (%) P No Yes

Gender , n(%)

Men	13(56,5)	10(43,5)	0,181
Woman	18(75)	6(25)	
Age, m±ET	40,77±12,16	40,75±17,32	0,996
(year)			

m: mean , n: number , SD: standard deviation

2.1.2. Comparison of clinical features:

The factors associated with the risk of digestive haemorrhage during follow-up were: digestive haemorrhage due to PH as the reason for discovery (22.2% in group 1 vs 77.8% in group 2) with a p value of= 0.004 and the presence of clinical signs of portal hypertension (37.5% in group 1 vs 62.5% in group 2) with a p value of $<10^{-3}$.

Table XI: Comparison of clinical features in the occurrence of gastrointestinal haemorrhage due to PH

Digestive haemorrhage n (%) P

	No	Yes	
Abdominal pain			
No	7(46,7)	8(53,3) 0,056	
Yes Digestive haemorrhage	24(75)	8(25)	
No	29(76,3)	9(23,7)	0,004
Yes AEG	2(22,2)	7(77,8)	
No	24(64,9)	13(35,1)	1
Yes Fever,	7(70)	3(30)	
No	30(67,7)	15(33,3)	1
Yes HVAC	1(50)	1(50)	
No	22(95,7)	1(4,3)	<10-3
Yes Jaundice	9(37,5)	15(62,5)	
No	27(65,9)	14(34,1)	1
Yes Splenomegaly	4(66,7)	2(33,3)	
No	24(88,9)	3(11,1)	<10-3
Yes Asymptomatic	7(35)	13(65)	
No	25(65,8)	13(34,2)	1
Yes	6(66,7)	3(33,3)	

AEG: impairment general condition , CVC: collateral venous circulation, n: number

2.1.3. Comparison of biological characteristics:

In univariate analysis, anaemia (p=0.014) and hyperleukocytosis (p=0.023) were factors associated with the occurrence of variceal haemorrhage.

Table XII: Comparison of biological characteristics in the occurrence of digestive haemorrhage due to PH

Digestive haemorrhage n (%) P No Yes

Cytolysis			
No	27(65,9)	14(34,1)	1
Yes	4(66,7)	2(33,3)	
Cholestasis			
No	23 (65,7)	12(34,3)	1
Yes	8(66,7)	4(33,3)	
BT(µmol/L)	17[10-25]	19[14,25-34,25]	0,216
BD(µmol/L)	4[2-9]	6[4-8,75]	0,223
Urea(mmol/L)	4,8[3,6-5,8]	3,46[4,45-6,9]	0,813
Creatinine(µmol/L)	65[56-72]	68[50-86,25]	0,946
Na(mmol/L)	137,32±2,94	137,31±4,58	0,993
K(mmol/L)	3,98±0,51	4,12±0,45	0,351
CRP(mg/L)	6[3-25]	5[2-19,25]	0,181
Hb(g/dL)	12,7[11,3-14]	10[8,7-12,5]	0,014
GB(elements /µL)	7196,54±2727,37	9201,25±2817,46	0,023
Platelets(elements /µL)	207000[138000-259000]	206000[171500-304000]	0,459

n: number

2.1.4. Comparison of imaging data

The presence of signs PH on imaging was associated with the risk of a digestive haemorrhage due to PH during follow-up (37.5% in group 1 vs 62.5% in group 2) with a **$p<10^{-3}$.** Extension to the mesenteric vein was not considered.

Table XIII: Comparison of imaging data in the occurrence of gastrointestinal haemorrhage due to PH

Digestive haemorrhage n (%)P NoYes

Extension to VMS			
No	21(65,6)	11(34,4)	0,944
Yes	10(66,7)	5(33,3)	
Collateral veins			
No	22(95,7)	1(4,3)	<10-3
Yes	9(37,5)	15(62,5)	
Splenomegaly No	24(88,9)	3(11,1)	<10-3
Yes	7(35)	13(65)	
Portal cholangiopathy No	27(65,9)	14(34,1)	1
Yes	4(66,7)	2(33,3)	

VMS: superior mesenteric vein , n: number

2.1.5. Comparison of endoscopic characteristics:

The presence of endoscopic signs of PH was associated with a higher risk of variceal haemorrhage during follow-up (48.3% in group 1 vs 51.7% in group 2).) with a p= 0.001.

Table XIV: Comparison of endoscopic characteristics in the occurrence of digestive haemorrhage due to PH

	Digestive haemorrhage	n (%)	P
	No	Yes	
Endoscopic signs			
PH			
No	17(94,4)	1(5,6)	0,001
Yes	14(48,3)	15(51,7)	
Grade of varicose veins Small	7(46,7)	8(53,3)	0,052
Big	0(0)	8(100)	

PH: portal hypertension , n: number

2.1.6. Comparison of treatment modalities :

Starting anticoagulant treatment was not associated with the risk of variceal haemorrhage during follow-up (p=0.069).

Table XV: Comparison of treatment modalities in the occurrence of digestive haemorrhage due to PH

	Digestive haemorrhage	n (%)	P
	No	Yes	
Anticoagulant treatment No	9(50)	9(50)	0,069
Yes	22(75,9)	7(24,1)	
n: number			

2.2. Multivariate study :

In multivariate analysis, the presence of endoscopic signs of portal hypertension (p=0.002) and the presence of collateral venous circulation imaging (p=0.014) were independently associated with the occurrence of variceal haemorrhage during follow-up.

Table XVI: Factors associated with the occurrence of digestive haemorrhage due to PH in multivariate analysis

	OR	IC95%	P
Endoscopic signs of PH	38,09	3,82-379,5	0,002
Collateral veins	19,15	1,79-204,3	0,014

PH: portal hypertension , OR: odds ratio , CI: confidence interval

DISCUSSION

In this chapter, we will analyse the main results of our study and compare them with those in the literature in order to identify the factors associated with the occurrence of haemorrhage due to PH. In our study, portal cavernoma was revealed by upper GI haemorrhage in 9 cases (19.1%). physical examination, clinical signs of portal hypertension: CVC and SMG, were the two most commonly reported signs present in 24 (51%) and 20 (42.5%) patients respectively.Liver function tests were normal in 75% of cases. The diagnosis was made by cross-sectional imaging with injection of contrast medium in all patients, showing total obstruction of the portal trunk with the presence a network of peri-portal and peri-cholecal collaterals forming the portal cavernoma.Extension to the VMS was detected in 15 patients (31.9%). A porto-systemic CVC and a GMS were present in 25 (53.1%) and 20 (42.5%) patients respectively. Signs of endoscopic PH were found in 29 patients (61.7%), 23 of whom had OV and 6 had hypertensive gastropathy.Anticoagulation was prescribed in 29 patients (61.7%). Mean follow-up was 52 months. A complication was noted in 24 patients (50.9%). Digestive haemorrhage due to rupture of the VO was noted in 16 cases (34%) with an average delay of 22.3 months. Of the 16 patients, 9 were taking VKAs. In 2 cases, digestive haemorrhage was responsible for death. Digestive haemorrhage due to PH was the leading cause of death in 2 patients.(4,2%). The analytical study revealed that the presence of endoscopic signs of PH (p=0.002; ORa=38.09; 95% CI [3.82-379.5]) and the presence of a CVC imaging (p=0.014; ORa=19.15; 95% CI [1.79-204.3]) were independent factors associated with the risk variceal haemorrhage during follow-up. The initiation of anticoagulant therapy was not associated with the occurrence of variceal haemorrhage.

1. PREVALENCE OF VARICEAL HAEMORRHAGE PATIENTS WITH PORTAL CAVERNOMA

Digestive haemorrhage due to PH is the most frequent complication during follow-up of patients with non-cirrhotic portal cavernoma. Its high morbidity and mortality make it a formidable complication (1). In our series, the rate of occurrence was 34% with an average delay of 20.4 months.The prevalence of GI haemorrhage due to PH varied between 28% and 35% according to the different studies, which is in line with our results (3,8). The study by Ferreira et al was carried out with the aim of establishing the natural history of PH and its complications in non-cirrhotic portal cavernoma. In this study, the natural history of VO appeared to be similar to that observed in patients with cirrhosis. In patients with no initial OVs, the risk of developing them was 2% at 1 year and 22% at 5 years. In patients with initially small OVs, the risk of developing medium or large OVs was 13% at 1 year and 54% at 5 years. In patients with medium or large OVs who received prophylaxis, the risk of bleeding was 9% at 1 year and 32% at 5 years (3). On the basis of this study, the Baveno VII consensus therefore recommends that EOGD be performed at the time of diagnosis of portal cavernoma and after one year'follow-up in the absence of VO (9-11).

2. FACTORS ASSOCIATED WITH THE OCCURRENCE OF GASTROINTESTINAL VARICEAL HAEMORRHAGE :

The study of factors associated with the occurrence of gastrointestinal haemorrhage due to PH in non-cirrhotic portal cavernoma was the subject of 4 studies: The study by Guillaume et al, carried out on 471 patients who underwent LEVO, showed no increased risk of haemorrhage in patients on anticoagulants during LEVO (12) . According to the latest Baveno VII conference, it is currently recommended not to stop anticoagulants and to LEVO in patients on VKA if the INR is within the therapeutic range of 2 to 3 (9). In the series by Amitrano et al (13), which included 121 patients with non-cirrhotic portal cavernoma, digestive haemorrhage occurred in 14 patients during follow-up (14.7%). Patients who initially presented with a variceal haemorrhage were more likely to develop one during follow-up (P<0.0001), which is in agreement with our results. In the series by Spaander et al, 43% of the 120 patients included developed GI haemorrhage due to PH, with an average delay of 7 months. Gastrointestinal haemorrhage at inclusion, the presence of ascites and initiation of anticoagulant therapy were identified as predictive factors for the occurrence of variceal bleeding during follow-up (14).

In another series involving 27 patients with non-cirrhotic portal cavernoma inaugurated by variceal haemorrhage, the risk of recurrence was 37%. Factors associated with haemorrhagic recurrence extension into the splenic vein and the presence of gastric varices on EOGD (15). In the series by Janssen et al , extension of the thrombosis to the superior mesenteric vein was the only factor associated with the occurrence of haemorrhage during follow-up (86)

.In the study by Ferreira et al, no predictive factor for the occurrence of variceal haemorrhage during follow-up was identified. The use of anticoagulants did not increase the risk of bleeding in patients with portal cavernoma. Furthermore, the risk of bleeding under primary prophylaxis with beta-blockers and of recurrence of bleeding under secondary prophylaxis were similar to those observed in cirrhosis (3). The first controlled trial evaluating the benefit of long-term anticoagulation in patients with non-cirrhotic portal cavernoma was conducted in 2022 by Plessier et al, and included 111 patients (55 on anticoagulants vs 56 without). This study showed that starting anticoagulants reduced the risk of thrombosis recurrence without increasing the risk of digestive haemorrhage due to PH(16) . Table XIX summarises the results of the various studies on the factors associated with occurrence of digestive haemorrhage due to HTP.

Table XIX: Factors associated with the occurrence of gastrointestinal haemorrhage due to PH reported the literature

Factors associated with	Amitran o	Spaande r	Jansse n	an d	Ferreira and	Our
occurrence of HDH	et al.(13)	et al(14)	al.(17)		al.(3)	study
by HTP	N= 121	N=120	N=119		N= 178	
						N=47
HDH as in circumstances of	+	+	-		-	+
discovery						
Signs of clinical PH	-	+	-		-	+
VO at EOGD	+	-	-		-	+
Anticoagulant therapy	-	+	-		-	-
Extension to VMS	-	-	+		-	-

HDH:upper gastrointestinal haemorrhage , PH: portal hypertension, EOGD: endoscopic oesophago-duodenal, VMS: superior mesenteric vein , N:number

11.STRENGTHS AND LIMITATIONS :

11.1. HIGHLIGHTS:

Non-cirrhotic portal cavernoma is a rare pathology. Our study is the first in Tunisia and in Africa to explore the complications of this pathology, mainly represented by HDH by HTP, by including a consequent number of patients compared to the studies reported in the literature. This was a study involving a group of patients with good follow-up and strict inclusion and exclusion criteria. As a result, the results were reliable and solid, consistent conclusions could be drawn.

11.2. Weaknesses :

Our study has a number of weaknesses, mainly due to methodological limitations. The retrospective and monocentric nature of our study are its main limitations.Data were collected from medical records. Consequently, there could be a selection bias. Some files were not included because they could not be used. Some of the data recorded lacked precision because they were collected from files in which the information sought could not always be found.

CONCLUSION

Non-cirrhotic portal cavernoma is a rare liver disease characterised by the formation of a network of portal collateral veins following obstruction of the portal trunk in the absence of underlying liver disease. The clinical picture is dominated by manifestations of portal hypertension. In view of the rarity of this pathology, the published data concerning the complications of portal hypertension are few in number. We proposed to carry out a retrospective cross-sectional study to evaluate the factors associated with the occurrence of digestive haemorrhage due to PH. Our study included 47 patients with non-cirrhotic portal cavernoma between January 2010 and December 2019 managed in the hepato-gastroenterology department at the Sahloul university hospital.

The mean age was 40.7 years with a sex ratio (male/female) of 0.95. A history abdominal surgery was noted in 8 patients (17%) with an average delay between diagnosis and surgery of 7.2 months. Porto-cava collateral venous circulation was present in 51.1% of patients and GMS in 42.5%. Liver function tests were normal in 75% of cases. The diagnosis was made by cross-sectional imaging with injection of contrast medium in all patients, showing total obstruction of the portal trunk with the presence of a network of peri-portal and peri-chole ductal collaterals forming the portal cavernoma.

Extension to the VMS was revealed in 31.9% of patients. A portosystemic CVC and a GMS on imaging were present in 53.1% and 42.5% of patients respectively. EOGD showed VO in 48.9% of cases and hypertensive gastropathy in 38.2%. Anticoagulation was prescribed in 61.7% of patients. Specific treatment for underlying diseases was instituted. After an average follow-up of 52 months, half of our patients (50.9%) presented at least one complication, dominated by digestive haemorrhage due to PH in 34% of cases. Digestive haemorrhage due to PH was the main cause of death in 2 cases. The aim of our analytical study was to identify the factors associated with the occurrence of digestive haemorrhage due to PH.

The factors associated with the occurrence of gastrointestinal haemorrhage due to PH in univariate analysis were: gastrointestinal haemorrhage as the reason for the discovery of portal cavernoma (22.2 % in group 1 Vs 77.8% in group 2 with a p = 0.004), the presence of clinical signs of PH (37.5% in group 1 Vs 62.5% in group 2 with a p **$<10^{-3}$**), the presence of anaemia (p=0.014) or hyperleukocytosis on laboratory tests (p=0.023), the presence of signs of portal hypertension on follow-up imaging (37.5% in group 1 vs 62.5% in the group with a **$p<10^{-3}$**) and the presence of endoscopic signs of PH (48.3% group 1 vs 51.7% in group 2 with a p=0.001).In multivariate analysis, the presence of endoscopic signs of portal hypertension (p=0.002) and the presence of collateral venous circulation on imaging (p=0.014) were independent factors associated with the occurrence of variceal haemorrhage during follow-up.

Anticoagulant treatment was not associated with an increased risk of haemorrhage during follow-up. These results allow us emphasise the importance of effective management of PH in non-cirrhotic portal cavernoma, especially when manifestations of PH are at the forefront, without delaying the possible initiation of anticoagulation. Our work revealed the factors associated with the occurrence of digestive haemorrhage due to PH during follow-up. Our results are consistent with those of various published studies. However, some of our significant results need to be put into perspective, given the small size of our sample and the single-centre nature of our study. Multicentre prospective studies are essential to confirm our results and establish clear recommendations.

REFERENCES

1. Debray D, Soret J, de FS, Raucourt ED. AFEF 2018 MVF RECOMMENDATIONS. 2018;25.

2. Balfour GW, Stewart TG. Case of Enlarged Spleen Complicated with Ascites, Both Depending upon Varicose Dilatation and Thrombosis of the Portal Vein. Edinb Med J. jan 1869;14(7):589-98.

3. Noronha Ferreira C, Seijo S, Plessier A, Silva-Junior G, Turon F, Rautou PE, et al. Natural history and management of esophagogastric varices in chronic noncirrhotic patients, nontumoral portal vein thrombosis. Hepatology. May 2016;63(5):1640-50.

4. Recommendations from the Baveno VII conference: Hepato-Gastro Oncol Dig. 1 Apr 2022;29(4):425-42.

5. Merkel C, Zoli M, Siringo S, van Buuren H, Magalotti D, Angeli P, et al. Prognostic indicators of risk for first variceal bleeding in cirrhosis: a multicenter study in 711 patients to validate and improve the North Italian Endoscopic Club (NIEC) index. Am J Gastroenterol. Oct 2000;95(10):2915-20.

6. Sarin SK, Lahoti D. Management of gastric varices. Baillieres Clin Gastroenterol. Sept 1992;6(3):527-48.

7. Primignani M, Carpinelli L, Preatoni P, Battaglia G, Carta A, Prada A, et al. Natural history of portal hypertensive gastropathy in patients with liver cirrhosis. The New Italian Endoscopic Club for the study and treatment of esophageal varices (NIEC). Gastroenterology. July 2000;119(1):181-7.

8. Condat B, Pessione F, Hillaire S, Denninger MH, Guillin MC, Poliquin M, et al. Current outcome of portal vein thrombosis in adults: Risk and benefit of anticoagulant therapy. Gastroenterology. Feb 2001;120(2):490-7.

9. de Franchis R, Bosch J, Garcia-Tsao G, Reiberger T, Ripoll C, Baveno VII Faculty. Baveno VII - Renewing consensus in portal hypertension. J Hepatol. Apr 2022;76(4):959- 74.

10. Sharma P, Mishra SR, Kumar M, Sharma BC, Sarin SK. Liver and Spleen Stiffness in Patients with Extrahepatic Portal Vein Obstruction. Radiology. June 2012;263(3):893-9.

11. Sarin SK, Gupta N, Jha SK, Agrawal A, Mishra SR, Sharma BC, et al. Equal efficacy of endoscopic variceal ligation and propranolol in preventing variceal bleeding in patients. with noncirrhotic portal hypertension. Gastroenterology. Oct 2010;139(4):1238-45.

12. Guillaume M, Christol C, Plessier A, Corbic M, Péron JM, Sommet A, et al. Bleeding risk of variceal band ligation in extrahepatic portal vein obstruction is not increased by oral Anticoagulation: Eur J Gastroenterol Hepatol. May 2018;30(5):563-8.

13. Amitrano L, Guardascione MA, Scaglione M, Pezzullo L, Sangiuliano N, Armellino MF, et al. Prognostic Factors in Noncirrhotic Patients With Splanchnic Vein Thromboses. Am J Gastroenterol. nov 2007;102(11):2464-70.

14. Spaander MCW, Hoekstra J, Hansen BE, Van Buuren HR, Leebeek FWG, Janssen HLA. Anticoagulant therapy in patients with non-cirrhotic portal vein thrombosis: effect on new thrombotic events and gastrointestinal bleeding. J Thromb Haemost. March 2013;11(3):452-9.

15. Spaander MCW, Murad SD, van Buuren HR, Hansen BE, Kuipers EJ, Janssen HLA. Endoscopic treatment of esophagogastric variceal bleeding in patients with noncirrhotic extrahepatic portal vein thrombosis: a long-term follow-up study. Gastrointest Endosc.May 2008;67(6):821-7.

16. General session I. J Hepatol. July 2021;75:S191-204.

17. Janssen H, Wijnhoud A, Haagsma E, van Uum SHM, van Nieuwkerk CMJ, Adang R, et al. Extrahepatic portal vein thrombosis: aetiology and determinants of survival. Gut. Nov 2001;49(5):720-4.

SUMMARY

Problem: *Chronic portal thrombosis outside the context of cirrhosis, also known as non-cirrhotic portal cavernoma, is a rare pathology of the liver characterised by the formation of a network of porto-portal collateral veins, the main manifestation of which is digestive haemorrhage due to portal hypertension.*

***Objectives**: The aim of our work was to identify the factors associated with the occurrence of digestive haemorrhage due to portal hypertension in non-cirrhotic portal cavernoma.*

***Methods**: We conducted a monocentric retrospective cross-sectional study in the gastroenterology department of Sahloul University Hospital over a 10-year period from January 2010 to December 2019. In order to evaluate the factors associated with the occurrence of GI haemorrhage due to portal hypertension, we divided the patients into 2 groups according to the occurrence of GI haemorrhage due to portal hypertension during the follow-up period. The various parameters (epidemiological, clinical, biological, radiological, endoscopic) were compared between the two groups.*

Results: *Our study included 47 patients with non-cirrhotic portal cavernoma. The mean age was 40.7 years, with a sex ratio (male/female) of 0.95. Abdominal pain was the most frequent symptom (68%). Porto-cava collateral venous circulation was present in 51.1% of patients and splenomegaly in 42.5%. The diagnosis was made by cross-sectional imaging with injection of contrast medium in all patients, showing total obstruction of the portal trunk with the presence a network of peri-portal and peri-cholecal collaterals forming the portal cavernoma. Extension to superior mesenteric vein* *was revealed in 31.9% of patients. Oeso-gastro-duodenal revealed oesophageal varices in 48.9% of cases and hypertensive gastropathy in 38.2%. 61.7% of patients were prescribed anticoagulation. Specific treatment for underlying diseases was instituted. After an average follow-up of 52 months, half of our patients (50.9%) presented at least one complication, dominated by digestive haemorrhage due to portal hypertension in 34% of cases. In the multivariate analysis, the presence of endoscopic signs of portal hypertension (p=0.002) and the presence of collateral venous circulation on imaging (p=0.014) were independent factors associated with the occurrence of variceal haemorrhage during follow-up. Starting anticoagulant treatment was not associated with an increased risk of haemorrhage during follow-up.*

Conclusion: *Non-cirrhotic portal cavernoma is a rare disease, most often affecting young adults. The clinical picture is dominated by complications of portal hypertension, hence the importance of effective management of its manifestations without delaying the possible initiation of anticoagulants. Therapeutic management remains a challenge for the clinician and must always be discussed in a multidisciplinary consultation meeting.*

TABLE OF CONTENTS

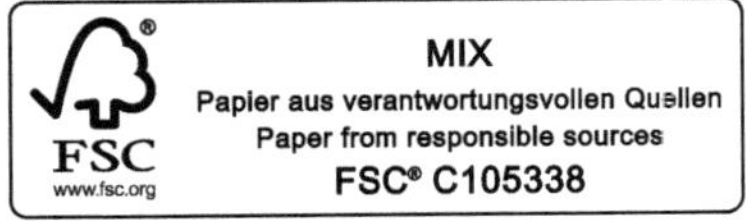

Printed by Books on Demand GmbH, Norderstedt / Germany